MW01277098

Everyone is talking

THE DIAGNOSTIC DILEMMA

"This book has concise information in an easy format that we all need either for ourselves or loved ones. Chapter One is outstanding!"

Dick and Kay Shaffer
Recovered brain surgery patient and wife

"**THE DIAGNOSTIC DILEMMA** is a helpful guide through the bewildering maze of medical diagnostic tests for patient and loved ones. It offers explanations, practical suggestions and personal experience as guiding lights to help anyone through the labyrinth of high-tech medicine with less stress and anxiety than would exist without it."

Reverend Bill Duckworth, Pastoral Care
First Presbyterian Church of Orlando, Florida

"This book does an excellent job of pointing out the various stages of an illness and the thoughts and feelings involved in those stages. As I recalled my recent health problems, I could relate to so much of what is in the book. It is a comfort to know that others going through a medical diagnostic process have similar thoughts and feelings. I highly recommend this book to patients, their families and friends."

Thomas C. Spear Jr.
Recovered pulmonary embolism patient

"I believe this book fulfills a need in the lay person by explaining in simple terms the medical diagnostic process."

Juan J. Herran, M.D., FCCP, FACP

"**THE DIAGNOSTIC DILEMMA** is an excellent book for patient, family and friends. I highly recommend it."

Sister Joanne Dewald OCD, M.S. Nursing
Carmelite Monastery, Indianapolis, Indiana

"Pam Melvin's real life experience produced a practical guide we can all use. She demonstrates how the diagnostic process builds character and allows one to find the real meaning of life."

Jewel Hodges
Husband of fibromyalgia patient

THE DIAGNOSTIC DILEMMA

*A Guide Through The Medical Diagnostic Process
For Patient, Family & Friends*

THE DIAGNOSTIC DILEMMA

A Guide Through The Medical Diagnostic Process
For Patient, Family & Friends

by

Pam Melvin

Milkovich Publishing Company

Book Design by Thistle Publications
Cover Design by Kitty Drybrough Shepherd
Index by Angela Washington-Blair, PhD.

Library of Congress Catalog Card Number: 96-94035

ISBN: 0-9649710-0-3

Printed in the United States of America.

Contents

Contents

Acknowledgements

*To my family and friends whose prayers, thoughts, and
comforting conversations sustained me throughout
my medical diagnostic process.*

❧

*To the Medical Professionals at the Mayo Clinic who
while practicing their respective areas of medical expertise
haven't lost sight of the human element.*

❧

*To Dr. Jack Baskin and Dr. Willard Boardman whose time,
advice and wisdom were unselfishly given to me
during my diagnostic dilemma.*

❧

*To Toni Pinzari whose advice as well as skill is exceptional
and will always be welcomed.*

❧

*To Lynne S. Bootay whose experience as a parent of a
child going through the medical diagnostic process prompted
the inclusion of a section on children as patients.*

❧

To C. J. Whiston, Jr. who always believed there would be a book.

❧

*To patients who are taking a more active role in their health care.
They are demanding to be treated with the respect and dignity
that should be afforded all human beings.*

❧

*To the couple I passed on the way to retrieve my
medical records at the pulmonary doctor's office.
Emerging from the elevator, x-ray envelope in hand,
the lady's eyes were filled and ready to overflow onto her face.
The gentlemen was patting her on the back,
saying it would be okay – a look of terror in his eyes.
Their identity was unknown;
however, what was known was the fear and uncertainty
they were both feeling as part of the
medical diagnostic process.*

Introduction

~

"I don't want to simply be a recipient
of all that is good in this life.
I want to give something back to
acknowledge my many blessings."

—Pam Melvin

I'd like to say that the idea for this book came to me at the moment I saw the couple exiting the elevator at the doctor's office, however, it was really the next morning as I waited for a plane to take me to Rochester, Minnesota and the Mayo Clinic.

I wondered — How could some good come from my medical diagnostic experience? What do I have in common with others who have gone through this process, are going through it now, or will go through it in the future? What could we use to help us through the process that isn't available today?

In this day and age, with increased disease and illness, most of us will experience a medical diagnostic process in our lifetime or that of a loved one. It can be a difficult process, regardless of the final diagnosis.

I believe there are tips / ideas / thoughts to be shared that might ease the burden, stress, anxiety, and sometimes the confusion of the process.

Not everyone is alike — so not everyone will experience the medical diagnostic process in the same manner. I believe, however, that there are enough similarities in all of us for the thoughts in this book to have some universal meaning and appeal — be it a sentence, paragraph or chapter.

This book is not intended as a substitute for medical advice and/or treatment. The reader should consult a physician in matters relating to his/her health.

Nor is this book intended to be the "gospel" on the subject. I am an expert only in that I've been both a family member of a patient, and a patient going through the medical diagnostic process.

As a family member of a patient, I participated in the process when my mother was diagnosed with colon cancer in April 1994. Surgery removed the cancer and part of her colon. Today, approximately one year later, she has completed chemotherapy and been told there are no additional tumors.

As a patient, I experienced the medical diagnostic process from the end of July through October 1994.

Upper back pain led me to an orthopedic doctor for what I thought would be a prescription for muscle relaxers. When my x-rays revealed a spot on my lung (described as a 6-8 centimeter liquid filled lesion that could be tuberculosis) and a need for a CAT scan, a pulmonary specialist, and a thoracic surgeon, my medical diagnostic process began.

The CAT scan was performed the next day. The radiologist's conclusion was metastatic disease from primary lung carcinoma.

The pulmonary doctor performed a transbronchial biopsy two days later to rule out carcinoma.

The biopsy was performed on a Friday and the results were available to me the next Tuesday in the doctors office — an anxious five days to say the least!

That Tuesday I heard the news that no malignancy was identified. The pathologist's report indicated "necrotizing granulomatous inflammation and fibrosis". The pulmonary doctor started me on medication for tuberculosis while acid fast bacilli cultures for the disease were being watched in a microbiology lab at the hospital. I was also sent to the hospital for blood work so that a fungal panel could be performed.

On subsequent office visits, I asked the pulmonary doctor what it could be, and was told several times — tuberculosis, a fungal infection, Wegener's, or (though highly unlikely) an old infection.

Perhaps it was a year of pre-med or my obsessive/compulsive nature, but I decided to do some research of my own and headed to the hospital library.

I wanted to find out more about Wegener's, which by now had been mentioned several times by the pulmonary doctor. When asked, his brief description consisted of: It is an autoimmune disease of unknown origin. It progressively attacks the body's organs and is not good if it goes to the kidneys. There is no cure and the treatment is steroids and chemotherapy. In other words, not something you wish for.

The library was full of reference materials on Wegener's Granulomatosis. What I read about the disease correlated with the medical problems I had experienced over the last four years: eye problems; a benign breast cyst; sinus problems; upper respiratory problems and finally a lesion in the lung.

The other striking feature of these articles was a continuing reference to the Mayo Clinic as a medical establishment that had experience treating this disease. What I later learned was that the medical professionals at the Mayo Clinic had seen about 500 cases of Wegener's since the 1950's.

As a result of my hospital library visit I was now anxious to get to the Mayo Clinic, but I wanted to "defect check" my thought process with two physicians whose opinions I respect. Both listened to my diagnostic process thus far — the fact that the biopsy was not malignant, the fungal panels were negative, and the tuberculosis cultures were negative. They agreed that going to the Mayo Clinic was an appropriate decision.

In mid August 1994 I flew to Rochester, Minnesota armed with physician reports about my sinus, breast, and eye problems as well as my most recent chest x-rays, CAT scan, and written pathology report from the transbronchial biopsy. I checked into the Mayo Clinic and began a diagnostic process which included physician consultations; blood tests; urine and stool tests; eye examinations; ear, nose and throat examinations; pulmonary tests; EKG; and chest x-ray.

The Mayo Clinic pathologists reviewed the biopsy report I had brought with me but also wanted to personally view the biopsy slides from the transbronchial biopsy I had in Florida. The slides were requested several times from a Florida hospital and once received and reviewed were felt to be inconclusive for Wegener's.

An open lung biopsy was discussed as a diagnostic tool to determine what was wrong with my lung. A thoracic surgeon reviewed my CAT scan and indicated:

- Because of the size and position of the lesions a larger incision would be necessary
- It would be known during surgery whether it was malignant or benign.
- Even though the pathology from the transbronchial biopsy indicated it was benign there was still a possibility that it could be lung cancer or lymphoma.
- If it was lymphoma they could begin chemotherapy treatments. If it was lung cancer there was not much they could do.

The surgery was performed on a Friday and I was told in the recovery room that it was not malignant.

The tissue samples were reviewed by three of their lung pathologists who indicated that the histologic features were most consistent with an infectious granulomatous disease. Cultures and microbiologic staining of the tissue samples removed during the open lung biopsy however have been negative.

While the clinical suspicion was consistent with a vasculitis, such as Wegener's granulomatosis, there has been no pathologic confirmation of that process.

So I'm being watched very carefully. Follow-up visits at the Mayo Clinic in Jacksonville, Florida have thus far been favorable.

Is my mother's bout with cancer or my experience with a lung disease unique? — I think not.

Similar instances of illness and disease are occurring all over the planet with increasing frequency.

This book exists to assist those patients, their families and friends as they travel through their medical diagnostic dilemmas.

Chapter 1

∾

THE PROCESS

"Diseases can be our spiritual flat tires —
disruptions in our lives that seem to be
disasters at the time, but end by redirecting
our lives in a meaningful way."

— Bernie S. Siegel, M.D.
Peace, Love & Healing

$\mathcal{T}$he medical diagnostic process can begin quite simply with an individual experiencing a symptom that they don't consider to be normal.

The symptom can be fairly recent — or, the symptom can be something that the patient has experienced for some time. The fact that it hasn't gone away, or has gotten worse, prompts action on their part.

The action is usually making a doctor's appointment.

In some cases, the process begins by a family member or friend who, after hearing about the symptom and discomfort of their loved one, either urges them to get medical attention or actually schedules the appointment.

Many diagnoses can be made by doctors during that appointment, treatment prescribed and the patient asked to follow up, depending on the diagnosis. In other cases, diagnoses can't be made without further testing. Depending on the nature and severity of what is probable, the process can become lengthy.

The duration is dictated by the number of tests / procedures that are deemed necessary, as well as the time frames for test results. The specific tests and time frames are detailed in Chapter Two.

As these tests / procedures are being performed, the process becomes a mix of what I call "active" and "non-active" time.

Active time is the time when the patient is "actively" involved in a test / procedure. Blood tests, biopsies, x-rays, CAT Scans, etc. are examples of active time.

Non-active time is time when you're waiting for results, waiting for the next test, waiting for a doctor's appointment, etc. It is a time without answers — and, while active time can be uncomfortable and sometimes painful because of needle pricks or endoscopes; it's the non-active time that is hardest from a mental perspective. This is covered in more detail in Chapter Three.

The medical diagnostic process can also begin as a result of an injury or condition that requires immediate or emergency care. Heart attacks, injuries sustained on the job or injuries as a result of accidents are examples. With these types of situations, the diagnostic process takes on a sense of urgency. Depending on the severity of a patient's situation, the process may begin in a doctor's office and be transferred to a hospital. In most cases, the process begins in a hospital emergency room.

Diagnostic tests / procedures are ordered on an emergency basis — and results are obtained on a priority basis.

Regardless of whether the process begins with a symptom or an injury; patients, family members and friends describe the process as:

- Frightening;
- Confusing;
- Cloaked in Mystery by the Medical Profession;
- Frustrating;
- A Roller Coaster;
- Filled with Time Delays;
- Overwhelming;
- Out of Control;
- Stressful;
- Emotionally Exhausting;
- Disheartening;
- A Waiting Game.

While this book doesn't claim to erase these thoughts in describing the process, it will provide you with some ideas or tips to help you and your loved one during the process.

The following ideas/tips are a compilation of my diagnostic experience, as well as the experience of other patients, family members or friends who were gracious enough to share their insights:

- As with all professions, there are degrees of expertise within the medical community. There are good doctors, great doctors and outstanding doctors. It's *your* life — Seek out the outstanding doctors!

- Get a second opinion. Physicians themselves, when faced with a diagnosis of cancer, get a second opinion, as well as a second pathologist to read their slides.

- You might say, "It's easy to say get a second opinion, but there's the issue of cost to the patient". In many cases, health care plans will pay for second opinions — and, for some procedures, the plans require it.

- Second opinions do require some work on the part of the patient. You need to find another physician (sometimes a specialist), arrange for an appointment, and, in some cases, provide your slides, x-rays or scans. This will add time to the process.

  Aren't you worth it! Think of the times when you've gotten multiple estimates before having something repaired (your car, roof, plumbing, etc.). Think of this in the same way — It's really the very least we can do for ourselves! I don't know about you, but I value my body more than the car, roof, or pipes in my house!

- As the patient, you should be straightforward with your doctor and as *proactive* as possible in your care. If emotionally you aren't up to the challenge, ask someone who is up to the challenge to do it for you! If you take only one thought from this book, take this one!

- Before you find yourself a patient going through a diagnostic process, determine and discuss this topic with a loved one—be that family or friend—who is capable and willing to be your support person. Discuss, in advance, what you see their role being and how you would like them to handle it. If they're not comfortable, give them the opportunity to tell you so... and move on to another person.

- Be prepared when you visit the doctor as a part of the diagnostic process. Formulate the questions you have—better yet, write them down. Let the doctor know up front that you have some questions to ask before the visit is concluded. And, most importantly, ask the questions! Some individuals prepare them, but become intimidated when they are with the doctor and never ask them.

- If you're not happy with your doctor and his/her approach to your health care, get another doctor! There are lots of physicians — and you deserve what you feel is the best for you! Let the physician know why you're unhappy and leaving their practice.

  A friend wrote a letter to a doctor and told him she wouldn't be back and why. In this particular case, she explained it was his coldness, unwillingness to answer her questions and the way he threw her file on the pile at the nurses station outside the examining room. She said she felt better for having written the letter, and added that perhaps it might alter his attitude toward his other patients.

- There are a number of ways to move on to another doctor in the medical community. Don't allow fear of not finding one to cause you to stay with someone who is less than satisfactory in your view.

- Ask other physicians/specialists that you regularly use to refer you — They're in the medical community and know which ones they or their family members would personally use.

- Call the local hospitals — Ask them which doctors have operating privileges at that hospital. If your situation is heart-related, ask about their cardiologists / thoracic surgeons.

- Nurses are an excellent source for referrals. In fact, some hospitals have services called "Ask A Nurse". You can receive information about local physicians — credentials such as schools, degrees, time in practice — by calling the service.

- If doctors are mentioned in newspapers/magazine articles for their work in a particular specialty, make a note — start a file.

- Use the book *The Best Doctors In America* by Steven Naifeh & Gregory White Smith or the excerpts from that book which were published in two consecutive 1995 issues of *Town & Country* magazine.

- Use a medical research service company like The Health Resource, Inc; 564 Locust Street, Conway, Arkansas 72032. (501) 329-5272.

- If you've used what you feel are the best resources locally and you're still in the medical diagnostic process, without answers — seek out a facility touted for its diagnostic abilities. They're listed frequently in national publications like *U.S. News & World Report* and *USA*

Today. They include: the Mayo Clinic, John Hopkins, Sloan-Kettering and M.D. Anderson Cancer Center — to name a few.

- If you decide to go to one of the large diagnostic centers after starting your diagnostic process locally, be aware that the doctors will want to see all your records — x-rays, CAT Scans, as well as biopsy slides — not just the written report.

- I learned the hard way and added about 3-4 days to my process simply waiting for the hospital in Florida to mail the biopsy slides to the Mayo Clinic. The Mayo doctors had to check at least three different times to find out the whereabouts of the slides. Why did they want the slides? Because they wanted their pathologists to view them. This is important when their doctors have much more experience with a disease than the local medical community.

- If your "gut" instinct toward a scheduled test/procedure is negative or you are uncomfortable, don't docilely agree to proceed with it without first voicing your concern and having it addressed.

Chapter 2

❧

MEDICAL DIAGNOSTIC TESTS

*"Wherever the art of medicine is loved,
there also is love of humanity."*

— Hippocrates
Aphorisms

*I*n order to reach a diagnosis, your physician needs information such as your medical history, your symptoms and a physical examination. Additionally he/she may order specific medical diagnostic tests/procedures to obtain more information about your medical condition.

This chapter will address those diagnostic tests by providing:

A. An overview of the types of available diagnostic tests;

B. Specific descriptions of 24 of the most commonly used diagnostic tests:

- The purpose of the test
- The actual test/procedure
- Preparation or special instructions to the patient
- What the patient can expect after the test (side effects of the procedure and any restrictions)
- Results

C. Time frames for test results

OVERVIEW OF THE TYPES OF
AVAILABLE DIAGNOSTIC TESTS

There are hundreds — perhaps thousands — of medical tests that can be used to assist the medical community in the diagnostic process.

Its common to hear diagnostic tests referred to as non-invasive and invasive.

Non-invasive tests are produced outside the body and give an indirect view of the body's interior. X-ray procedures and sonograms are examples.

Invasive procedures require going into the body to view organs as well as take tissue samples or biopsies for further study. Transbronchial biopsies and sigmoidoscopies are examples.

Whether the tests are invasive or non-invasive, the more common tests include:

- Urine Tests
- Blood Tests
- Microbiological Tests
- Imaging Tests
- Nuclear Medicine Scans
- Endoscopic Tests
- Electrical Tests

URINE TESTS

Most complete medical exams include urine testing. It is used to test for glucose (sugar), ketones, protein or bilirubin in the urine. Since these substances aren't normally found in a person's urine, their presence is an indication that a disease may be present. The process involves either spontaneous collection (urinating into a container) or catheterized collection.

BLOOD TESTS

Complete medical exams also include blood tests. Like urine tests, blood tests are used to rule out or confirm diseases such as anemia, leukemia, lymphoma or infection.

The most common blood tests are:

- Complete Blood Cell Count (CBC)
- Blood Chemistry Group
- Lipids
- Erythrocyte Sedimentation Rate
- Thyroid Studies

Drawing blood is a relatively quick procedure that can be performed at a doctor's office, a laboratory or a hospital. Some blood tests require fasting prior to the test, while others do not. Your physician will instruct you if fasting is necessary.

MICROBIOLOGICAL TESTS

If a physician suspects the presence of a microorganism, he/she may order cultures of tissue or body fluid.

Cultures (the process of growing microorganisms in a laboratory for futher analysis) are used to identify the cause of infections, fungal diseases and tuberculosis.

The cultures do need time to produce/grow enough organisms to be identified — and this can take weeks, or even months.

Throat cultures and spinal taps are examples of these types of tests. They are used to diagnose strep throat, meningitis and infections of the central nervous system.

BIOPSIES

Biopsies are the removal of tissue samples for microscopic study. These samples are used to confirm or rule out diseases.

Tissue can be removed from the body using a knife, a needle or an instrument called an endoscope (see endoscopic tests).

IMAGING TESTS

Imaging tests use x-ray or other technology to create an image of the inside of the body. While traditional x-ray is still used for such tests as dental x-rays and mammograms, technological advances have led to the use of other methodology — namely, the use of computerized scanning equipment.

The most common scanning tests are:

- Computerized Tomography — or CT
- Magnetic Resonance Imaging — or MRI
- Ultrasonography

NUCLEAR MEDICINE SCANS

This process produces pictures of internal organs with the help of radioisotopes which are swallowed by or injected into the patient. These scans are used to help diagnose diseases of the liver, gallbladder and thyroid.

ENDOSCOPIC TESTS

Endoscopic tests fall in the category of invasive tests and are designed to examine the body's interior through the use of a rigid or flexible tube connected to an optical system.

This technology allows medical specialists to diagnose a wide variety of illness/disease. Some examples are:

Endoscopic Procedure	View Of:
Cystoscopy	Urethra & Bladder
Gastroscopy	Esophagus, Stomach & Duodenum
Bronschoscopy	Trachea & Bronchial Tree of Lungs
Arthroscopy	Joints
Laryngoscopy	Larynx
Sigmoidoscopy	Rectum & Sigmoid Portion of the Large Intestine
Colonoscopy	Lining of the Colon from the Anus to the meeting of the Small and Large Intestine

ELECTRICAL TESTS:

Our bodies produce electrical currents. Scientists have devised ways to monitor this electrical activity and study it in the diagnostic process.

Some of the common electrical tests are:

ECG (ELECTROCARDIOGRAPH): Measures the heart's electrical impulses and is used to diagnose heart damage, heart irregularity, or the effectiveness of heart pacemakers.

EEG (ELECTROENCEPHALOGRAPH): Measures the electrical activity of the brain and is used to diagnose seizure disorders.

EMG (ELECTROMYOGRAPH): Measures the electrical discharges produced by muscles and is used to diagnose muscle or nervous disorders, such as muscular dystrophy and ALS.

SPECIFIC DESCRIPTIONS OF 24 OF THE MOST COMMON DIAGNOSTIC TESTS/PROCEDURES

Some of the most common or most frequently ordered tests/procedures are described on the following 35 pages. The descriptions follow a similar format in providing the reader with:

- The purpose of the test
- Details of what happens during the test/procedure
- Preparation or special instructions to the patient
- What the patient can expect after the test (i.e. side effects of the procedure and any restrictions)
- Results

Three excellent and more detailed reference books on medical tests/procedures are:

The Patients Guide to Medical Tests by Cathey and Edward R. Pinckney

Medical Tests and Diagnostic Procedures by Philip Shtasel

Mayo Clinic Family Health Book by Mayo Foundation for Medical Education & Research.

Procedure: **ARTHROSCOPY**

PURPOSE: To view the interior of joints (knees, shoulders, etc.). Doctors can examine the tissue, as well as take a biopsy specimen or perform minor surgery.

PROCEDURE: The arthroscope uses an optical system to view the interior of joints. Either a local or general anesthesia is administered before a small incision is made and the arthroscope inserted. The doctor can then view via TV monitor the inside of the joint. This procedure usually takes about an hour.

PREPARATION: The patient is told not to eat or drink approximately 12 hours prior to the procedure.

FOLLOWING TEST: The joint undergoing the procedure will be swollen for several days and therefore should not be used for intense physical activity for several days.

RESULTS: Due to the fiberoptic equipment, visual results are known immediately by the doctor performing the procedure. Tissue samples (biopsies) are sent to a lab for analysis and generally take 3–5 days for results.

Procedure: **BARIUM X-RAY**

(Also known as an Upper-Gi Series/
Barium Milkshake and a Barium Enema)

PURPOSE: These two tests use x-ray and barium liquid to
view the upper and lower digestive tracts.
Abnormalities such as colon cancer, ulcers,
tumors, Crohns disease and ulcerative colitis
can be detected through these procedures.

PROCEDURE: **UPPER GI SERIES:**

The patient lies behind equipment called a fluo-
roscope. A milkshake-type drink of barium is
given to the patient to drink and he/she may be
asked to drink more of the mixture as the procedure continues. The patient may be asked to
change his/her position as the test is administered.

BARIUM ENEMA:

Again, the patient lies on a table behind the flu-
oroscope. A lubricated enema tip is inserted into
the rectum and a liquid barium mixture is
released into the bowel. The patient must
remain still and hold his/her breath as the x-rays
are taken — and the technologist will assist in
this regard. After a series of x-rays is completed,
the patient is allowed to go to the bathroom and
expel the barium. In some cases, the colon is
inflated with air and additional x-rays taken.

PREPARATION: **UPPER GI SERIES:**

The patient is told not to eat, drink, chew gum or — in some cases smoke — after midnight the night before the procedure. Teeth can be brushed, but do not swallow the water. The patient may also be asked to clear out the lower digestive tract with the help of a laxative.

BARIUM ENEMA:

For this test to be successful, the lower digestive tract must be clean. Therefore, preparation includes laxatives, enemas and suppositories, as well as restricting all food and drink. Solid food is usually stopped 2 days before the test.

FOLLOWING TEST: The barium in both the milkshake and the enema is passed out of the body in the stool. Often, a laxative is prescribed after a barium enema to be sure the barium leaves the body. For several days after the test, the stool may be light brown or white. Drink plenty of fluids after the procedure is completed. This will assist in the passing of the barium.

RESULTS: A radiologist will study the results of these procedures and provide an evaluation to your physician. These results are usually shared with the patient during a follow up visit with the doctor.

Procedure: **BRONCHOSCOPY**

PURPOSE: To view the inside of your lungs. Physician can look for abnormalities such as tumors of the lungs and airways.

PROCEDURE: Using an instrument called a bronchoscope, the doctor inserts it through the mouth or nose into the lungs. The scope contains a mechanism that produces an enlarged picture of the passageways of your lungs. The doctor can view this as the procedure takes place, as well as after the procedure is completed.

This procedure is generally performed in the hospital, and the patient is usually lying down. It is usually performed under local anesthesia, but can be performed under general anesthesia. The anesthesia depresses your cough and swallowing reflexes and is usually administered in both the nose and mouth.

PREPARATION: Patient will be told not to eat anything for 8–12 hours before the test.

BRONCHOSCOPY CONTINUED

FOLLOWING TESTS:

After the test, the patient should not ingest anything for about one hour because his/her reflexes are still depressed due to the anesthesia. Patients are also told not to drink alcohol or drive for 24 hours after the procedure. It is normal after the procedure for the patient to cough up some blood. However, if the amount of blood is excessive, the doctor should be called.

RESULTS:

Due to the fiberoptics of this procedure, visual results are immediately available to the doctor. Tissue or fluid samples (biopsies) taken during the procedure will be sent to a laboratory and usually take 3–5 days for results to be known.

Procedure: **CARDIAC CATHETERIZATION OR CORONARY ANGIOGRAPHY**

PURPOSE: To assist in the diagnosis of a heart problem. Viewing the inside of the heart and arteries assists in determining if the blood vessels are clogged; if the heart is pumping normally; if blood is flowing correctly and if problems were present at birth.

PROCEDURE: The patient is usually admitted to the hospital on the day of the procedure. Medication to help relax or sedate the patient may be administered, but the patient will remain awake. The skin where the catheter is inserted (arm or groin) is shaved. A long flexible tube or catheter is inserted into a blood vessel and guided by the physician to the heart. An x-ray screen shows the physician the movement of the catheter. Dye is injected along the catheter which helps identify any blockage that exists. Another x-ray (ventriculography) allows the heart's pumping activity and chambers to be viewed.

PREPARATION: The patient is instructed not to eat or drink anything after midnight the night before the catheterization.

CARDIAC CATHETERIZATION OR
CORONARY ANGIOGRAPHY CONTINUED

FOLLOWING
TESTS:

Once the tests are finished, the doctor removes the catheter from either your arm or groin. Several stitches may be used if the catheter was inserted in the arm. If it was inserted in the groin, that area will be pressed firmly for about 15 minutes to stop any bleeding. Usually a pressure bandage is placed on the insertion site which should not be moved for 4–6 hours. During this time the patient remains lying down. All of the above are done to prevent bleeding.

RESULTS:

Results are known during the procedure. These are used by your physician to decide if you need treatment and what is the best course of action. Generally this information is shared with the patient before release from the hospital or during a follow up visit with the physician.

Procedure: **COLONOSCOPY**

PURPOSE: Using a fiberoptic scope, the colon is viewed and examined. This procedure can detect polyps, cancer and other diseases of the colon.

PROCEDURE: Sedatives are generally administered intravenously to relax the patient prior to the beginning of this procedure. The patient is lying on his/her side on the examining table. A lubricant is applied around the anus and a colonscope is inserted into the rectum and large intestine, thus giving doctors a direct view of the lower gastrointestinal tract. Visual results that would indicate the presence of polyps or tumors can be determined during the procedure, due to the fiberoptic equipment.

PREPARATION: Patient must closely follow dietary restrictions and instructions for several days before the procedure. The night before, the patient must use a laxative. The morning of the procedure, the patient will have an enema to make certain the colon is as cleaned out as possible. A clean colon enables the fiberoptic equipment to get the best pictures of the colon.

COLONOSCOPY *CONTINUED*

FOLLOWING TEST:
Since the patient has worked to cleanse the colon for the procedure, regular bowel habits could be impacted. Drinking plenty of water is always good advice where bowels are concerned. Patient is advised to avoid any activity which requires alertness (driving or operating heavy machinery) due to the sedatives which have been administered.

RESULTS:
Due to the fiberoptics, visual results are immediate. Tissue samples that are removed for biopsy will generally take 3–5 days to analyze and produce results.

Procedure: **COMPUTERIZED TOMOGRAPHY OR CT SCAN / CAT SCAN**

PURPOSE: Using x-rays, the CT Scan produces three dimensional, cross-sectional images of the inside of the body. The process is considered better than a conventional x-ray in viewing internal structure. The most frequently conducted scans are body CT and head CT. These are used to assist in the diagnosis of brain disorders as well as kidney, lung, liver and pancreas problems.

PROCEDURE: The patient (in hospital gown) is positioned on a table that is moved through the CT scanner. The scanner is a large round machine with an opening in the center. It is through this opening that the patient is moved while x-rays are being performed. The patient must remain still during the process which generally takes 45 minutes to 1 hour. The patient may also be injected with or drink an iodine containing fluid that highlights the area to be x-rayed. This produces more defined images of the area in question. The images are viewed on a video screen during the procedure and photographs are made for the radiologist to read and analyze. During the process you may hear noise from the CT scanner. This is normal.

COMPUTERIZED TOMOGRAPHY OR
CT SCAN / CAT SCAN CONTINUED

PREPARATION: The patient should not eat for four hours prior to the procedure. If the patient knows he/she is allergic to iodine or seafood he/she should tell his/her physician before he/she is scheduled for the CAT Scan.

FOLLOWING TEST: After the procedure the patient may be asked to remain on the table while the radiologist examines the images and makes certain he/she has all the information needed to assist in the diagnosis. If this is the case the patient will be helped off the table, told to get dressed and resume normal daily activities. If a contrast medium fluid was administered, the patient may experience diarrhea.

RESULTS: The radiologist will analyze the CT images and send a report to your primary physician or the physician who ordered the test. Those results are generally discussed with the patient during a follow up visit with his/her doctor.

Procedure: **CYSTOSCOPY**

PURPOSE: To view the inside of the bladder and examine the urethra. Doctors can look for problems such as infection, cancer or chronic inflammation.

PROCEDURE: The cystoscope is a narrow fiberoptic tube that is inserted into the bladder. This instrument is designed to remove tissue, if necessary, so that a biopsy can be performed. Due to the fiberoptics, the doctor can view the bladder while the scope is being performed. Patients are generally given a local anesthesia for this test and remain awake.

PREPARATION: None.

FOLLOWING TEST: If a local anesthetic is administered, there are no restrictions. If a general anesthetic is used, the patient should rest after the procedure and not use alcohol or drive for 24 hours. There could be some urinary burning and/or slight bleeding after the procedure. Sometimes antibiotics are prescribed.

RESULTS: Due to the fiberoptics, some of the results are immediate. If tissue samples are taken for biopsy, the results could take 3–5 days.

Procedure: **DILATION & CURETTAGE (OR D&C)**

PURPOSE: Can determine the cause of frequent menstrua-
tion or heavy bleeding. It can also be used to
identify polyps, cancer or fibroids. Also used for
termination of pregnancy or following miscar-
riages.

PROCEDURE: Once dilated, the cervix allows an instrument
called a curette to scrape the uterine lining.
Current methodology also uses low pressure
suction to remove endometrial tissue. The
process can be done with a local anesthetic in a
doctor's office or under general anesthetic in a
hospital.

PREPARATION: Patient should not eat or drink for 12 hours
prior to procedure.

**FOLLOWING
TEST:** Patient is usually released from the hospital the
day the the procedure. She may experience
some pain and vaginal bleeding. For 24 hours
after the procedure, the patient should not drink
alcohol or drive. Tampons should not be used
for several weeks nor should sexual activity
occur for several weeks.

RESULTS: Visual results are known by the physician
immediately following the procedure. Biopsy
results will take 3–5 days.

Procedure: **ECHOCARDIOGRAM**

PURPOSE: To view the heart in action without using an invasive procedure. Using sound waves, the physician can view valves, veins and arteries to diagnose such things as coronary artery disease, blood clots or aneurysm.

PROCEDURE: Patient is positioned on his/her back. A special gel is applied to the chest and a transducer instrument is rubbed over the chest to produce images which are monitored on a screen.

PREPARATION: None.

FOLLOWING TEST: No aftereffects are noted.

RESULTS: The use of sound waves to produce images on a monitor screen allows the physician to have immediate test results. The images will also be studied after the procedure is complete.

Procedure: # ELECTROCARDIOGRAM (EKG) – EXERCISE OR STRESS TEST

PURPOSE: To determine if coronary artery disease exists. The procedure, through the use of exercise, increases the heart muscle's demand for blood. Whether this increased demand can be satisfied is monitored. If it can not, an inadequate blood supply exists.

PROCEDURE: Disks or electrodes are placed on the patient's shoulders, arms and chest. These electrodes are connected to wires that lead to an electrocardiograph machine. The patient is asked to step onto a treadmill or stationary bike and begin exercising. As the exercise becomes more strenuous, the patient's heart rate increases. His/her vital signs (blood pressure and pulse) as well as the electrocardiographic tracings are observed for symptoms. This procedure generally takes about one-half hour.

PREPARATION: The patient is given specific instructions which include: not eating or smoking prior to the test; avoiding some medications; and wearing comfortable shoes and clothing.

ELECTROCARDIOGRAM (EKG) — EXERCISE OR STRESS TEST
CONTINUED

FOLLOWING   Symptoms experienced during this test will
TEST: determine what the patient will be directed to
                   do by his/her physician.

RESULTS: Some results are known during the test, how-
                   ever, it is likely the patient's entire series of diag-
                   nostic tests will be reviewed by the physician
                   and discussed with the patient during a follow-
                   up consultation.

Procedure: # ELECTROCARDIOGRAM (EKG) – RESTING

PURPOSE: To view the electrical activity of the heart. Used to detect heart disease or specific heart problems.

PROCEDURE: The resting EKG requires the patient to lie motionless on his/her back on a bed or examination table. Pads or disks about the size of quarters are temporarily attached to the patient's skin on his/her chest, arms and legs. These disks lead to wires or electrodes that are connected with the machine which registers your heart's electrical activity. There is no discomfort associated with this test which lasts approximately 15 minutes.

PREPARATION: No preparation is needed.

FOLLOWING TEST: The disks/pads are temporarily affixed to the skin with the help of a lubricant. This substance is wiped off the patient's skin. Some patients may experience redness or tenderness of the skin where these disks have been affixed.

RESULTS: The machine is actually analyzing the electrical activity of the heart and recording it in the form of a graph as the test is being conducted. The results are known immediately.

Procedure: **GASTROSCOPY**

PURPOSE: To view the upper portion of the digestive tract (esophagus, stomach and duodenum). Allows physician to examine the interior of this tract, as well as remove tissue/fluid samples for biopsies.

PROCEDURE: Patient is lying down on his/her side. A local anesthetic is sprayed into the mouth and throat to suppress the patient's desire to gag. A sedative can also be administered. The doctor inserts a fiberoptic instrument through the mouth into the esophagus, stomach and duodenum to view these structures.

PREPARATION: Patient must fast for 8–12 hours prior to examination.

FOLLOWING TEST: If a sedative is administered, the patient should restrict his/her driving for 24 hours.

RESULTS: Visual results are immediate due to direct observation. Biopsies will be sent to laboratories for analysis and generally take 3–5 days.

Procedure: **INTRAVENOUS UROGRAPHY (OR IVU)**

PURPOSE: An x-ray examination which provides detailed pictures of the kidneys, ureters and bladder. This procedure is conducted if abnormalities are suspected such as tumors, stones, etc.

PROCEDURE: The patient is positioned on a table under a piece of x-ray equipment. A special medication will be injected into a vein. While this is happening, the patient may feel warm and flushed. Some individuals indicate there is a metallic taste in their mouth. This should only last for a short time and is no cause for alarm. If the patient begins to itch or feel short of breath, they should let the technician know. While the x-rays are being taken the patient may be asked to assume different positions.

PREPARATION: The patient will be instructed about specific fluid intake and diet that should be followed one or two days before the test occurs. Generally, six hours before the test, he/she must stop all intake of food and drink. A laxative, suppository or enema may be used to clean the bowel and thus provide a better view of the urinary tract.

INTRAVENOUS UROGRAPHY (OR IVU) CONTINUED

The patient should alert the technician who will perform the procedure if he/she have any allergies — specifically to seafood, codeine or radiologic contrast agents if they've had procedures where contrast medium has been used.

FOLLOWING TEST: There should be no aftereffects.

RESULTS: A radiologist will analyze the x-rays and report his/her findings back to the doctor who ordered the test. These results are reviewed with the patient during a follow up visit with his/her physician.

Procedure: **LAPAROSCOPY**

PURPOSE: Provides a view of a woman's reproductive organs. Assists in the detection of cancer, endometriosis, pelvic disease and ectopic pregnancy.

PROCEDURE: Patient will be given either a local or general anesthetic. Gas is inserted into the abdomen via an incision and needle. A fiberoptic tube called a laporoscope is then inserted and the inside of the abdomen is examined. Once the scope is removed, the small incision is closed by several stitches. Tubal ligation also can be performed during this procedure.

PREPARATION: Patient is instructed not to eat or drink for 12 hours before the procedure.

FOLLOWING TEST: The patient will generally have abdominal pain, due to the gas and procedure. This dissipates after several days. Most women indicate they want to take it easy for several days following the procedure.

RESULTS: During the procedure the uterus, tubes and ovaries can be scrutinized. The photographs produced by the fiberoptics equipment are analyzed by specialists and results given to the patient during a follow-up visit to the doctor.

LARYNGOSCOPY

Procedure: **LARYNGOSCOPY**

PURPOSE: To view the voice box or larynx to rule out problems such as a tumor or an abnormality.

PROCEDURE: A local anesthetic is sprayed into the nose and throat of the patient and suppresses his/her desire to gag. A fiberoptic instrument is inserted through the nose into the throat to view the larynx.

PREPARATION: The patient must fast for several hours before the test.

FOLLOWING TEST: The patient may experience some soreness in his/her nose or throat and could cough up a little blood. Food or drink should not be consumed until the anesthetic wear off – usually a half hour.

RESULTS: The use of fiberoptics provides some immediate results for the physician. Tissue samples will be analyzed in the laboratory and generally take 3–5 days to produce results.

Procedure: **LIVER BIOPSY**

PURPOSE: To diagnose liver disease or the progress of liver disease. The procedure can determine disorders such as hepatitis, tumors or cirrhosis.

PROCEDURE: The patient lies on his/her back and is given a local anesthetic to prevent discomfort. The doctor will insert a needle between or below the ribs into the liver and remove a tissue sample (biopsy) for analysis in the laboratory.

PREPARATION: Patient may not have anything by mouth after bedtime the night before the procedure.

FOLLOWING TEST: There could be some pain/discomfort or even bleeding after the procedure. As a result you will be monitored for several hours before you can go home. Patient should "take it easy" for several days following the visit.

RESULTS: Due to the need for the tissue sample to be analyzed in a laboratory results are usually known in 3–5 days.

MAGNETIC RESONANCE IMAGING (MRI)

Procedure: **MAGNETIC RESONANCE IMAGING (MRI)**

PURPOSE: Using magnetic fields and radio waves, the procedure provides detailed images of your body's internal structure. It is felt to be clearer than x-ray and does not use radiation like x-ray and CT scans.

PROCEDURE: The procedure is non-invasive. A technologist will position you on a padded table that electronically moves through a piece of equipment that resembles an enormous block with a hole in the center. The procedure itself is painless, but you will be asked to remain perfectly still throughout the exam. Depending on the type of MRI being performed, the test could take 45–90 minutes to complete, so this is a relatively long time to remain perfectly still. During the exam, the machine will make noise which has been described as a clanking or tapping sound. This is normal.

PREPARATION: The magnetic field may affect metallic devices, so you will be asked whether you have a pacemaker, have any implanted mechanical or electrical devices, have had a mitral or aortic valve replacement, brain aneurysm clips, a history of shrapnel or metallic fragments, or an optic implant.

MAGNETIC RESONANCE IMAGING (MRI) CONTINUED

You may eat and drink before the exam with no restrictions and should take prescribed medications.

You should not bring metal objects into the exam room, such as pocket lighters, hair pins, jewelry, partial plates for your mouth, dentures or hearing aids.

Wigs and eye makeup may interfere with brain MRIs. You should also indicate if you have permanent facial makeup (eyeliner, etc.) which has been tattooed on the skin and could contain metal.

FOLLOWING TEST: You can continue normal activities after the procedure is completed. If medication is administered to allay anxiety it's a a good idea not to drive immediately following the procedure.

RESULTS: The scans are read by an MRI specialist who is a physician trained in the specialty of radiology. Results are delivered to the doctor who scheduled the procedure and will be discussed with the patient during a follow up visit at the doctor's office.

MAGNETIC RESONANCE IMAGING (MRI)

MAMMOGRAPHY

Procedure: **MAMMOGRAPHY**

PURPOSE: Used to detect breast lumps/abnormalities that are so small they are not visible to the human eye or to touch. This procedure's effectiveness is increased when it is combined with regular breast exams and regular self-examinations.

PROCEDURE: Low doses of x-rays produce images of the inside of the breast. The patient may be asked to sit or stand. Compression of the breast is necessary and is generally done by a plastic shield. Several x-rays will usually be taken of each breast.

PREPARATION: Patient will be told not to use deodorant, powder or perfume in the breast or underarm area. Since you'll undress from the waist up, it is advisable to wear a blouse or sweater.

FOLLOWING TEST: The radiologist will check the x-rays and determine if more are necessary. The patient may have some breast tenderness after the procedure.

RESULTS: X-rays are analyzed by a radiologist and compared to previous mammograms. Results are generally given to patient at conclusion of the procedure. If an abnormality is noted or there is an unclear picture, the procedure may be followed with a sonogram.

Procedure: **NUCLEAR MEDICINE SCANS**

PURPOSE: Use of a special camera and a liquid that is swallowed or injected allows internal organs to be viewed. Diagnoses such as thyroid tumor; liver tumor or gallbladder disease can be made.

PROCEDURE: The patient lies on a special table under a piece of equipment called a gamma camera. A radioactive material is either injected into the patient's vein or swallowed by the patient. This radionuclide travels through the bloodstream to the organ in question. The gamma camera will take several images of that organ. Either the camera will be rotated or the patient is asked to assume several different positions on the table. During each scan or image the patient will be asked to lie still. The procedure can last 30 minutes to several hours, depending on the organ being scanned.

PREPARATION: Depending on the type of scan, the patient may be asked not to eat or take medication before the procedure. Metallic objects such as jewelry should be removed.

FOLLOWING   No special care is required.
TEST:

NUCLEAR MEDICINE SCANS *CONTINUED*

RESULTS: Nuclear scans are performed by trained technologists and analyzed by physicians. Results are usually ready the day of the procedure, however, the nuclear medicine physician will discuss findings with the patient's doctor who ordered the test. Results are discussed with the patient during a follow up consultation with his/her doctor.

Procedure: **OPHTHALMOSCOPY**

PURPOSE: To view the back of your eye and examine the blood vessels, retina and optic nerve. This procedure can provide information to assist in evaluating eye disorders.

PROCEDURE: Drops are placed in the patient's eyes to dilate the pupils. This enables more of the back of the eye to be seen. An instrument called an ophthalmoscope shines a light through to the back of the eye and the physician can clearly examine the eye.

PREPARATION: The patient's eyes will be dilated by drops and the examining room lights will be dimmed in an effort to have the pupils as wide as possible.

FOLLOWING: It takes some time for the pupils of the eyes to
TESTS: return to normal size. They will be light-sensitive and this may interfere with one's ability to see clearly. Sunglasses should help reduce the sensitivity to light.

RESULTS: Results are immediately known by the physician performing the test. They are generally shared at that time with the patient.

PAP SMEAR

Procedure: **PAP SMEAR**

PURPOSE: To detect precancerous conditions or cervical cancers at a stage when they cannot be viewed without a microscope.

PROCEDURE: Performed during a woman's pelvic examination. An instrument, inserted by the doctor, scrapes the surface of the cervix, removing cells which are then placed on glass slides and sent to a laboratory for examination under a microscope. The woman is positioned on a table with her feet in stirrups and her legs bent at the knees. In this position, the doctor can perform the Pap smear, as well as the pelvic exam.

PREPARATION: None.

FOLLOWING TESTS: Woman may experience some sensitivity and slight bleeding.

RESULTS: Since the tissue/cell samples must be observed under a microscope, the results are not immediate. Most laboratories indicate Pap smear results are available in 6–8 days. New procedures are reducing this time frame and a national laboratory now indicates they can provide Pap smear results in 3–4 days.

Procedure: ## PROCTOSIGMOIDOSCOPY (PROCTO)

PURPOSE: Used to examine the interior of a portion of the colon (rectum and sigmoid), as well as obtain tissue samples for biopsy. This procedure is used to screen for colon cancer, as well as diagnose Crohn's disease or ulcerative colitis.

PROCEDURE: Patient lies on table, usually on his/her side, while physician inserts a fiberoptic instrument called a protosigmoidoscope in the patient's rectum. This equipment permits the physician to examine the rectum and lower colon.

PREPARATION: Patient must prepare his/her bowel by administering enemas prior to the procedure.

FOLLOWING TEST: No restrictions are noted. There may be some bloating or cramping for several hours after the exam.

RESULTS: The use of fiberoptic equipment provides some immediate results to the physician. Tissue sample will be sent to a laboratory for biopsy and take longer to produce results.

TONOMETRY

Procedure: **TONOMETRY**

PURPOSE: Used to measure the ocular pressure or pressure
                 within the eye, and thus indicate the possibility
                 of glaucoma.

PROCEDURE: There are several types of tonometry tests being
                 used: the air-puff tonometer; Schiotz tonometer;
                 and the applanation tonometer. The most com-
                 mon of these administered by an ophthalmolo-
                 gist is the applanation tonometer. The eyes are
                 anesthetized with drops and, while the patient is
                 sitting, the equipment is placed directly against
                 the eyeball. The device denotes eye pressure.

PREPARATION: Eyes are anesthetized with drops.

FOLLOWING   The patient's eyes may feel scratchy as the
TESTS: anesthesia wears off.

RESULTS: The tonometer produces immediate results for
                 both physician and patient.

Procedure: ## ULTRASONOGRAPHY (SONOGRAM)

PURPOSE: Uses sound waves to capture images of internal
                organs. These images are displayed on a video
                screen during the test and made into photo-
                graphs which can be studied after the procedure
                is completed. A variety of organs can be studied
                this way: kidneys, liver, bladder, and female
                reproductive organs. The two most common
                sonograms are pelvic and abdominal.

PROCEDURE: ### PELVIC SONOGRAM

                The patient is asked to remove his/her clothing
                and put on a hospital gown. A table that resem-
                bles a bed is used and the patient rests on his/her
                back. Oil or gel is applied to the pelvic area by a
                technician who then passes an instrument called
                a transducer over the oiled area. This allows a
                good contact to be made between the skin and
                transducer and ultimately better pictures of the
                internal organ(s).

                Before the test proceeds, the technician will pass
                the transducer over the bladder to see if it is full
                enough. This is important because a full bladder
                helps push the bowel away from the organs to be
                viewed. If the bladder is not full enough the pro-
                cedure may not proceed until the patient drinks
                additional water. Once the technician verifies

ULTRASONOGRAPHY (SONOGRAM) CONTINUED

that the bladder is full enough the test will continue. During the procedure the patient is asked to remain still and to occasionally hold his/her breath.

Patient discomfort is common because of a full bladder. Once the test images are felt to be complete the patient is helped off the table and allowed to empty his/her bladder.

ABDOMINAL SONOGRAM

Most of the above steps apply; however, there is no need for a full bladder. The transducer, when passed over the skin, will produce light pressure. With the abdominal test, the patient may be asked to turn on his/her side or stomach.

In both examinations, once the test is complete, the oil or gel is wiped off the abdomen/pelvis. These examinations generally take less than an hour. A bladder that is not full could cause the pelvic test to take longer.

PREPARATION: **PELVIC SONOGRAM**

The patient is asked to drink a large quantity of water before the exam is performed. It is important that he/she refrain from urinating until the doctor/technologist indicates that he/she can do so.

ULTRASONOGRAPHY (SONOGRAM) CONTINUED

ABDOMINAL SONOGRAM

Preparation begins the day before the test and can include diet, laxatives and medication designed to clean the bowel. Patient is instructed to fast (no food, drink or chewing gum) 12 hours before the exam.

FOLLOWING
TESTS:

There are no aftereffects to the abdominal sonogram. The patient will feel relief, once he/she is allowed to urinate after the pelvic sonogram. He/she may find that they need to empty their bladder more than once following the exam.

RESULTS:

PELVIC SONOGRAM

The use of ultrasound technology provides immediate results for the radiologist, obstetrician or gynecologist conducting the test. The images gathered from the procedure can also be analyzed after the test.

ABDOMINAL SONOGRAM

Again, the sound wave technology known as ultrasound or sonogram allows some results to be known to the radiologist during the exam. The images that are produced can also be evaluated after the procedure is completed.

Generally, the radiologist reports findings of your scan to your physician.

TIME FRAMES FOR
TEST RESULTS

Earlier in this Chapter, the statement is made that the timing of test results varies according to the methodology of the procedure and what analysis is necessary.

Results are known during the actual procedure in some instances. Fiberoptics have enabled the physician to transfer images of the body to a screen for viewing during the procedure, as well as produce still photographs for additional analysis.

Other tests, such as biopsies and blood work, can require analysis by pathologists or hematologists and increase the time frames for results.

While this is true, there are some usual and customary time standards that the medical community subscribes to and the patient, as the user of these services, should know what they are. In doing so, they equip themselves as more knowledgeable patients.

In researching the issue of time frames for test results, an international laboratory, a national laboratory, all the local hospitals and several independently-operated radiology facilities were contacted.

It should also be noted that the larger medical diagnostic establishments, such as the Mayo Clinic, perform their diagnostic tests/procedures within their own facility and have the most expedient time frames for results. This can diminish the anxiety of patients, their friends, and family.

Each facility, be it independent laboratory, hospital laboratory, etc., will tell you that they establish their own time frames for test results.

Remember that they are often in competition with each other, so you're not likely to find wide variations on what they can deliver to their customer.

Likewise, laboratories pride themselves on accuracy and this is one of their selling factors. However, laboratories are also dealing with the human element, and mistakes can be made.

There is mention elsewhere in this book of a need for second opinions. The potential for errors in test results is one reason for obtaining them.

I like to think of the total time frame for test results as having six key elements or components:

1. ### SCHEDULING OF THE TEST/PROCEDURE:

    This is generally done by a member of the physician's staff and is predicated on availability. While the doctor may wish the procedure to be done as soon as possible, the next available opening may be days or weeks away. If this happens and you are concerned about the waiting period, ask if there are alternative facilities to be used for the procedure.

2. ### PREPARATION TIME FOR THE TEST/PROCEDURE:

    Specific preparation time is detailed earlier, as a part of the description of the **24** most common diagnostic tests. They generally begin 1–2 days in advance of the procedure/test and are dietary restrictions and/or intestinal cleansing.

3. ### THE TIME IT TAKES FOR THE ACTUAL TEST/PROCEDURE TO BE PERFORMED:

    Procedures vary in the length of time they take to complete. Some are as quick as 10–15 minutes (Pap Smear), while other can take an hour or more.

4. **THE TIME IT TAKES THE DATA TO BE REVIEWED &**
   ANALYZED (*X-RAYS, CT SCANS, MRI's, BLOOD WORK,*
   ***TISSUE SAMPLES, ETC.*):**

   These time frames also vary by type of test and, therefore, type
   of data. The usual time frames for the categories of tests are:

TEST CATEGORY	USUAL TIME FRAME
Blood Tests (CBC) (Sedimentation Rate) Most Thyroid Tests	**24 Hours** *(Laboratory to Doctor's Office)*
Biopsies	**3–5 Days** *(Laboratory to Doctor's Office)*
Pap Smears	**7–8 Days** *(Laboratory to Doctor's Office)*
Microbiology	**24 Hours Preliminary Results; 48 Hours for Final Results** *(Except Cultures, such as Tuberculosis, which can take Weeks or Months)*
Sonograms CT Scans MRI's Upper & Lower GI's	**24–48 Hours** *(Laboratory to Doctor's Office)*

These time frames will continue to improve as medical technology is enhanced. While researching this issue, a national laboratory indicated that their new pap smear procedure produces
results in 3–4 days versus the traditional 7–8 days.

5. TRANSPORT OR TRAVEL TIME

This is the time it takes for the data (blood, tissue, fluid, CT scans, MRI's, X-rays, sonograms) to be transported from one location to another.

If the test is performed in the doctor's office and data needs to be analyzed in a laboratory (the doctor's office doesn't have one), this is the time it takes data to be sent to the lab and returned from the lab to the doctor's office.

If the procedure is performed in a hospital and data analyzed in their laboratory, the transport time is the time it takes for data to travel from the hospital to the doctor's office.

If the procedure is performed at an independently-operated facility, the transport time is the amount of time it takes for the results to be sent to the office of the doctor who ordered the procedure.

The methods of transport are continually being improved and, with today's technology, they include: mail service; courier; telephone and fax machine; on-line printer and on-line computer access.

Many of the larger laboratories offer on-line computer and printer access to doctors' offices as a way of expediting the time frames for results.

The type of results can also dictate the way they are transported. CT scans can't be faxed and are generally couriered or mailed. The radiologist's analytic report of those CT scans can be faxed.

It's also not uncommon, in the case of x-rays, MRI's, CT scans and ultrasounds, for the patient themselves to transport or courier them from the facility where they were performed to the doctor's office.

The contractual agreement a doctor's office has with a laboratory can also impact the overall time frames for transport. Some agreements stipulate one daily lab pick-up, while others state multiple daily pick-ups.

6. **THE TIME ESTABLISHED FOR PATIENT'S FOLLOW-UP VISIT WITH THE PHYSICIAN:**

   This visit is traditionally used to communicate test/procedure results to the patient, as well as discuss appropriate courses of action based on the results.

   This appointment, usually scheduled by the doctor's staff during the patient's previous visit, allows enough time for the test results to be received by their office, as well as coordinate with the doctor's schedule.

   Results are sometimes shared via telephone, but most are shared in person. Of course, the exception to this is a patient whose diagnostic tests require hospitalization and who is still hospitalized when the results are communicated.

Delays can and do occur during any of the six components. My own diagnostic process contained an example of these delays...

On 8-2-94 I had blood drawn at a local hospital for a fungal panel. On 8-15-94 the doctor indicated he did not have any results from this fungal test. That same day I inquired at the hospital if results were available and was told that they had been mailed on 8-8-94 to the doctor.

When I asked whether I could get a copy of the results which had been mailed to the doctor I was told that they would make them available to me as long as I signed a release. Armed with that information and the directions to the hospital laboratory, I knew on 8-15-94 that the results from the fungal panel were negative... something the pulmonary doctor said he couldn't tell me on that same date!

While I'm not advocating that this is the proper way for the patient to receive test results, it is a vehicle available to the patient when the traditional process doesn't appear to be working.

The lesson I learned from this incident is have your laboratory work when possible performed at a hospital facility and not the doctor's office. Not everyone would agree with this — definitely not doctors who are equipped to perform tests in their office and want to do so to help defray the expense of their equipment.

Unfortunately, my experience with a test result delay is not unique. While I believe it is the exception and not the rule, people have started sharing their stories with me.

One in particular comes to mind... A mammogram was performed late in the day on 12-16-94. No radiologist was available to read and analyze the report and the patient was told the results would be mailed to her physician. As of 12-27-94 the patient had heard nothing and called the facility where the mammogram was performed. They indicated the report was mailed on 12-20-94, and that she should follow up with her doctor. On 12-28-94, the patient called the doctor's office and was told by an office staff member that the results had been received but with the holidays they had neglected to call her. Much later that day, the physician called and indicated the results were okay. Eight working days transpired before the patient received results that were available on 12-19-94, one working day after the test was performed.

Chapter 3

❦

The Patient

*The more serious the illness,
the more important it is for you to fight back,
mobilizing all your resources—
spiritual, emotional, intellectual, physical.*

— Norman Cousins

*I*f you are a patient going through the medical diagnostic process, I believe your body, mind and spirit will be impacted. Most of the scientific community already acknowledges that these three human dimensions play an important role in leading a healthy life. Likewise, they are impacted as you experience a medical diagnostic process. While not everyone will experience the same combination of the three, there are many similarities for all of us.

YOUR BODY

The patient's physical body is usually the first component of the mind/body/spirit connection to be impacted during a medical diagnostic process. It is generally the reason you are involved in the process to begin with. There is a physical discomfort or pain; a body part hurts; a system (digestive, cardiovascular) isn't working. In other words, a symptom that something is physically out of sync.

So your body is giving you a signal. A signal you should heed by contacting a physician and starting the process.

If you have been treating your body well (proper diet and exercise) you should continue to do so.

If you haven't been treating your body properly, try to change those habits and incorporate good nutrition and exercise into your life. Of course check first with your physician. In most cases he/she will recommend you do so.

Keeping your physical strength up throughout the diagnostic process is important. There will be times when your emotions will interfere with your appetite or interest in your physical appearance.

Remember that the body/mind/spirit are important in balancing the healthy human being.

Don't be afraid to do things for your physical self:

- Ask for hugs often;
- Have a partner/loved one give you a back rub;
- Have your feet massaged;
- Determine your favorite exercise and start doing it;
- Make a concerted effort to eat healthier foods.

YOUR MIND

Just as you fuel your physical body with food, your thoughts fuel your mind. During a medical diagnostic process these thoughts seem to take on a life of their own. It is without question an emotional time. The duration of the process as well as the diagnosis and treatment generally dictate the life cycle of these thoughts.

Diagnostic processes of a short duration such as waiting several days for a test result, still have an impact on your mind. Processes that require longer time frames (weeks and even months) can be mental/emotional roller coasters for both patients and their loved ones.

Fear, anxiety, despair (call it what you want), can become your unwelcome visitor. Its hard to get this house guest to leave. While it is never welcome, it will try to stay as long as possible. You must decide when these thoughts/emotions should leave and there are ways to help them pack their bags.

When you can't sleep at night and you lie there thinking of worst case scenarios, fear will spread itself a gourmet meal on your bed and have a feast with your every thought! Send those thoughts packing by getting up and doing something!

- Read a book. Perhaps one of the self-help books mentioned in Chapter Six will help you focus on positive thoughts.
- Listen to self-help tapes or your favorite music.
- Turn to your spiritual side through prayer or reading the Bible. There are specific verses and prayers for those who can't sleep:
  2 Samuel 22:29
  2 Corinthians 4:6
  Psalm 31:1-5
  Matthew 11:28-30
  Job 11:17
  Psalm 4:8
  Philippians 4:6-7
  John 8:12

- If physical activity keeps unwanted thoughts at bay then participate in that activity — clean, wash clothes, cook, paint, garden, exercise — Do what works for you!
- Talk to a family member or friend. One of my friends offered to be available at any time to talk and she meant it!
- If writing your thoughts in a journal appeals to you – do it! It can be very cathartic. In fact both patient and their loved ones can keep journals that capture their thoughts and feelings. Sometimes it's easier to write these down than talk about them. The journals might also become the basis for conversation that otherwise would be difficult to initiate.

A friend told me about his mother. She had fear and depression as her constant companions during a lengthy medical diagnostic process. They had lived on a farm years ago and he felt she would relate to an analogy using that experience. He related that he asked her to remember the farm and specifically the old dog they had on the farm. He reminded his mother that when that dog had nothing to do it dug holes everywhere. He told his mother that was what she was doing — mentally digging holes. As corny as it sounded, he said it helped her to diminish the fear and depression.

Understand that as you go through this process you may want help in dealing with your emotional state. Family and friends may not be equipped to deal with this aspect. Even if they are equipped, they may not be the right individuals to turn to for help.

Seek professional help. See a counselor or join a support group. All communities have these resources available. If you don't know how to access them, call the Mental Health Department, United Way, employee assistance program at your employer, or local churches for referrals.

Patients also can have a tendency during a diagnostic process to become somewhat self-centered and/or withdrawn. I believe this is the body's natural defense mechanisms at work. However, for loved ones this can be disturbing and is often misunderstood (more on this in Chapter Four Family and Friends).

There is a psychological phenomenon called "shut down" or ceasing to listen to shocking news, that can happen to patients during the process. I call it going "numb and dumb". It can happen to anyone during the process. Family and friends are not exempt from this either.

Let me give you a personal example. During a day of multiple medical procedures, an EKG technician indicated to a group of us that we should get undressed from the waist up and put the green gowns on in preparation for our EKGs. No sooner had she given the instructions than I started to take off my slacks. When they hit my ankles, I thought to myself – I don't think my heart is down here and quickly pulled them up before anyone realized what I had done.

YOUR SPIRIT

If your spirituality is intact and strong, you already know how important this aspect is during a diagnostic process. It sustains you. It can help diminish your anxiety or keep fear totally at bay. It's your best companion during the fitful, sleepless hours.

If you've been in spiritual limbo — or totally void of any spiritual dimension in your life — Change that!

RUN, don't walk — to your nearest church, rectory, synagogue, parish, temple or house of worship.

Have no guilt feelings about doing so — GOD is delighted to have you back. He is much more forgiving of you than you are of yourself.

If you feel guilty, seek out a religious individual to discuss this. If you don't know how or where to start the process of contacting someone in the clergy, think of someone whose spirituality you admire and ask that person to help you with setting up an appointment. They will be happy to do so.

While visiting a house of worship, see what written materials are available. While at the Mayo Clinic, I frequented a historic Episcopal Church that had numerous pamphlets and literature for visitors. Pamphlets such as these were extremely helpful to me:

- Why Do People Suffer?
- Be Of Good Cheer
- Prayers For the Middle Of The Night
- Before Your Operation
- Healing Everywhere
- How To Pray
- What Is Faith?
- Dealing With Our Doubts

The majority of these are available through Forward Movement Publications – 412 Sycamore Street, Cincinnati, Ohio 45202.

It's interesting to note that, regardless of the outcome of medical diagnostic processes, patients continually proclaim their illnesses or diseases as "gifts". For many of these individuals, their diagnoses are life-threatening: cancer, MS, lupus — yet they are unwavering in their convictions.

You can travel through a diagnostic process on a purely scientific basis — but, the body, mind and spirit are a powerful combination that will enrich your life.

CHILDREN AS PATIENTS

Thus far the use of the word "patient" has been an adult reference. Perhaps it is our desire to protect children that causes a natural inclination away from considering them as patients. Unfortunately they are not exempt from medical diagnostic processes.

With help from a friend and parent of a child who experienced a lengthy medical diagnostic process the following thoughts are offered.

- Depending on the child's age, involve them when possible in the process. Older children should feel they are participating and have a degree of control over their situations.

- Acknowledge the child's symptoms and also his/her fears.

- If the child has observable symptoms — keep track of the time, frequency, and duration. Better yet, videotape the symptoms for viewing by the physician. That way if the symptoms are not present on the day of the doctor appointment, he/she will have some visual evidence of what the parent and/or child is trying to describe.

- If a child is scheduled for tests/procedures, try to explain what is going to happen in terms they can understand. The medical community has expertise in doing this — make sure they use it!

+ Parents know their child much better than anyone else. If the child continues to exhibit symptoms or complains that something is wrong and you as the parent instinctively feel that something is not right about your child's health, don't let the medical establishment try to tell you otherwise. It may be that a doctor doesn't have the expertise in a particular field that is necessary for the diagnosis.

+ Use any of the tips mentioned in Chapter One to help locate a doctor and/or medical establishment that can help your child.

The July 24, 1995 issue of *U.S. News & World Report* lists the top hospitals for pediatric care.

Chapter 4

❧

FAMILY & FRIENDS

"Nobody can do it alone.
We all need the loving support of family
or a caring friend."

— Robert H. Schuller
God Is Good

*J*ust as you can travel through a medical diagnostic process on a purely scientific basis, you can also experience the process without the support of family and friends.

But, this is NOT recommended!

Some individuals, for a variety of reasons, have a solitary experience — and, while it can be done, the process is enriched by the involvement of your loved ones.

In this book, the terms loved ones and family and friends are synonymous — and, I believe, they can be defined as people who care about a patient going through a medical diagnostic process.

Family and friends can be emotionally impacted by what the patient is going through and experience some of the same feelings that the patient does.

Fear, anxiety about test results, and terror at potential relationship changes dictated by medical conditions are some of the emotions that can be experienced by loved ones.

While feeling a range of emotions, family and friends have another important role to assume — support for the patient.

So theirs is a dual role — dealing with their own emotional response to the situation, while providing support for the patient.

Often times this is complicated by a patient that appears to be withdrawing from his/her support — and/or loved ones who are uncomfortable with their support role to the point of absence.

Let's talk first about the patient who is focusing inwardly, as a result of the body's natural defense mechanisms.

For family and friends, this can be disconcerting and mis-understood. Loved ones may feel that the patient is pushing them away or rejecting them because of something they've said or done and start to second-guess their actions. This only adds undue strain to an already emotional situation.

Be knowledgeable in the potential for this to occur.

My advice: Give the patient space to focus inwardly, but let them know you're there for them, care for them and will do whatever they want or need you to do. You can't, however, read their minds — so, they must let **you** know what **they** want or need! Sometimes, the message is subtle — and, as family or friend, you'll need to discern what is being said or not said.

I remember gathering my dirty clothes together in the hotel room where a friend and I were staying during my visit to the Mayo Clinic. The friend sensed the need I had, saw it as a way she could help and picked up my clothes and headed to the laundry room. By doing so she was satisfying two of my needs — clean laundry and providing me some time alone.

Sometimes, it will require you to ask the patient what you can do for them. Be prepared for their response to include, "I don't know" or "leave me alone". Believe the first; ignore the second! Don't leave them alone, in the figurative sense. They may, however, be telling you they literally need some space. In your desire to help them, you may be overbearing — and this is their way of letting you know.

I mentioned earlier in this chapter, that relations between patient and loved ones could be complicated by a patient withdrawing, or family and friends' discomfort with the situation. The discomfort that family and/or friends feel can come from various sources:

- Being scared of the diagnosis;
- Being terrified of mortality — the patient's or their own;
- Not knowing what to say to a patient;
- Afraid they'll say something wrong or stupid;
- Afraid they won't be able to handle their own emotions;
- Afraid the patient won't be able to handle his/her emotions.

Whatever the reason, try to remember that this is a time when family & friends are desperately needed. Patients need to know you're thinking about them. They don't need to hear you say anything philosophical or profound... they just need to hear your voice.

Juliet Wittman in her June 1993 *Glamour* magazine article *How To Be A Good Friend To Someone Who's Ill* said it best: "A little bit of sensitivity — a genuine effort to understand — can make all the difference. A simple, "I heard what you've been going through" will suffice. After that, you can take your cue from the patient. They may seize the opportunity to discuss everyday things or treatment options. Despite my annoyance at some friends' dismissive or thoughtless remarks, I generally found even the clumsiest attempts at comfort, even the worst verbal blunderings far less hurtful than silence.

When family and friends are comfortable with the situation, their care and concern for the patient can take many forms — all of which are appreciated:

- ◆ Listen to the patient! If your conversation with the patient has been primarily one-sided — with you listening and the patient talking, and sometimes incessantly — you're on the right track.

- ◆ Allow the patient to repeat things in conversation, without pointing it out to them. This happens because they don't remember that they've said it... or because talking about the situation helps them to handle it. In most cases, it's the latter — so, listen as if you're hearing it for the first time.

- ◆ Don't attempt to diminish what the patient is feeling by getting them to focus on other thoughts or by changing the topic of conversation.

- ◆ If you can make and keep the commitment, offer to be available any time to talk. A wonderful friend said that I could call her any time during the night when I couldn't sleep. That meant a lot — and I knew she was sincere!

- ◆ Let the patient freely express his/her emotions about the situation with you. Give them a safe haven to cry. Likewise, let them vent their anger/frustration. Another friend of mine knew this instinctively and said to me during one of my weepier moments when I was apologizing for tears: "Don't ever say you're sorry for crying with me. Friends share good times as well as tough times with each other."

• Be tolerant of changes in the patient's views on life. Many individuals going through the process become more spiritual. Don't criticize a person's thoughts or feelings in this regard.

• It's okay for family and friends to show emotion with an individual going through the medical diagnostic process. Contrary to what some feel is a non-supportive act, it may be the ultimate act of care and concern letting them know you share in their pain.

• Offer the patient transportation to their doctor appointments, diagnostic tests and/or hospital appointments.

• Offer the patient transportation to establishments that will help meet their daily needs, i.e. grocery store, bank, post office, etc.

• Offer to run errands for them — pick up prescriptions. The offers of transportation are also somewhat safety-driven. Going through a diagnostic process can have the effect of keeping you preoccupied — a mental state which doesn't mix well with operating a vehicle.

• Sometimes *don't* offer, just *do* something for the patient!

• Invite the patient out for a meal. It's a great way to personally assure that he/she will at least eat properly at that time!

• Hug them... hold their hand. Most people today are starved for some physical contact. If you're not sure how they would react to a hug, saying something like: "I'd like to hug you — would that be okay?" will answer the question for you.

- Don't offer your advice regarding aspects of the process, unless it is asked for, or you believe the patient is making decisions that have the potential to do harm.

- Be reassuring — but not phony. It's reassuring to hear someone say, "Whatever the diagnosis, we will tackle this together — I'll be there for you."

- Send greeting cards. Decide whether humorous or serious greetings are appropriate.

- Handwritten letters and notes are almost a lost art. It was very touching to me to know someone took the time to send me a personal message.

- Send gifts that are uplifting or inspirational. I received a book titled, *Poems Of Joy & Hope*, that I've read several times.

- There are times during the process when some pampering would be welcomed: a facial, massage, pedicure, manicure, day of beauty — are all things that a patient isn't apt to have as a priority. In fact, some of the things a patient routinely does to enhance his/her appearance will be of less importance during this time. That's why some pampering can be both mentally and physically uplifting.

Chapter 5

GIFTS FROM THE PROCESS

"Thank you God for healing,
for new life and real hope
when I thought there was none."

— Greg Anderson
Healing Wisdom

*R*egardless of the outcome of the diagnostic process, patients continually proclaim their illness and/or the processes involved as "gifts"! You might say... sure, for anyone who comes out of the process with good news they have every reason to rejoice and be euphoric. But the patients that proclaim their "gifts" have oftentimes been diagnosed with life threatening illnesses.

Bernie Siegel, M.D. in his book *Peace, Love and Healing* says it best. "They understand that illness can help heal their lives, that it can bring new meaning to relationships with lovers, family and friends. That doesn't mean they don't wish to be well, but that they wouldn't give up what they have achieved because of their illness."

My "gifts" were numerous during my two and a half month medical diagnostic process and they continue today. They include:

* Realization of the joy of my friendships.

- A Mayo Clinic nurse who reached across the desk and held my hand when things got tough.

- Strengthening a childhood friendship through similar diagnostic processes.

- An astute clinical psychologist who helped me listen to and speak from my heart.

- Physicians who were secure enough in their professions and beliefs to say "We don't have all the answers".

Think of your "gifts" as you travel through the medical diagnostic process. Record them if you like in the space below.

Chapter 6

A Reading List

*W*ithin many books are thoughts and statements that can be extremely meaningful to individuals — be they patient, family or friend — going through the medical diagnostic process.

While they helped me tremendously once I sought them out during my process, I would encourage you not to wait until you're in the midst of a diagnostic dilemma to read them.

Most bookstores carry the books I have listed or can order them. Public libraries are also an excellent source. The list is not intended to be all-inclusive, but should get you started!

The list begins with the **Holy Bible** and is followed by books listed alphabetically, by author.

AUTHOR	BOOK TITLE
Allen, Charles L.	*God's Psychiatry*
Anderson, Greg	*Healing Wisdom*
Cousins, Norman	*Anatomy of an Illness as Perceived by the Patient*

COUSINS, NORMAN . . . . . .*The Celebration of Life*

DOSSEY, M.D., LARRY . . . .*Meaning & Medicine*

DOSSEY, M.D., LARRY . . . .*Healing Words*

GRAHAM, BILLY . . . .*Hope For The Troubled Heart*

HAY, LOUISE . . . .*Heal Your Body*

HAY, LOUISE . . . .*You Can Heal Your Life*

HIRSHBERG, CARYLE &
BARASCH, MARC IAN . . . .*Remarkable Recovery*

LE SHAN, LAWRENCE . . . .*How To Meditate*

MOYERS, BILL . . . .*Healing & The Mind*

NAPARSTEK, BELLERUTH . . .*Staying Well With Guided Imagery*

NAIFEH, STEVEN &
SMITH, GREGORY WHITE . .*The Best Doctors In America*

ORNSTEIN, ROBERT &
SOBEL, DAVID . . . .*The Healing Brain*

PECK, M.D., M. SCOTT . . .*The Road Less Traveled*

PECK, M.D., M. SCOTT . . .*Further Along The Road
Less Traveled*

ROUD, PAUL . . . .*Making Miracles*

SCHULLER, ROBERT . . . . .*Life's Not Fair, But God Is Good*

SCHULLER, ROBERT . . . . .*Tough Times Never Last,
But Tough People Do!*

SIEGEL, M.D., BERNIE . . . .*Love, Medicine & Miracles*

SIEGEL, M.D., BERNIE . . . .*Peace, Love & Healing*

SIEGEL, M.D., BERNIE . . . .*How To Live Between Office Visits*

SIMONTON, M.D., O. CARL *Getting Well Again*

STEARNS, ANN . . . .*Living Through Personal Crisis*

WEIL, ANDREW . . . .*Spontaneous Healing*

Copyright
Acknowledgements

❧

Bibliography

Anderson, Greg. *Healing Wisdom*. New York: Penguin Books USA Inc., 1994

Cousins, Norman. *Head First, the Biology of Hope*. New York: E. P. Dutton, a division of Penguin Books USA Inc., 1989.

Griffith, H. Winter. *Complete Guide to Symptoms, Illness & Surgery*. New York: The Putnam Publishing Group, 1989.

Krames Communication. *Understanding Body CT*. California: Krames Communication, 1985.

Krames Communication. *Abdominal Sonogram*. California: Krames Communication, 1984.

Krames Communication. *Pelvic Sonogram*. California: Krames Communication, 1985.

Krames Communication. *Understanding Magnetic Resonance*. California: Krames Communication, 1985.

Krames Communication. *Stress EKG*. California: Krames Communication, 1984.

Krames Communication. *Nuclear Medicine Scans*. California: Krames Communication, 1983.

Krames Communication. *Upper GI Series*. California: Krames Communication, 1984.

Mayo Foundation for Medical Education and Research. *Mayo Clinic Family Health Book*. New York: William Morrow and Company, 1990.

Miner, Margaret and Rawson, Hugh. *The New International Dictionary of Quotations-Second Edition*. New York: Dutton, an imprint of New American Library, a division of Penguin Books USA Inc.,1986,1993.

Pinckney, Cathey and Edward R.,M.D. *The Patient's Guide to Medical Tests*. New York: Facts On File Publications, 1978, 1982, 1986.

Rosenfeld, M.D., Isadore. *The Best Treatment*. New York: Simon & Schuster, 1991.

Schuller, Robert H. *God is Good*. Tennessee: Thomas Nelson Publishers, 1993.

Shtasel, Philip. Medical Tests and Diagnostic Procedures: *A Patient's Guide to Just What the Doctor Ordered*. New York: Harper & Row, Publishers, Inc., 1990.

Siegel, Bernard S. *Peace, Love and Healing*. New York: Harper & Row, Publishers, Inc.,1989.

Index

A

B

C

G

Gallbladder

  nuclear medicine scan of, 45

  ultrasonography of, 51

Gamma camera, 45

Gastroscopy, 17

  description and details, 36

Glaucoma, 50

Glucose, urine testing for, 14

God, importance of Him in diagnostic process, 68

Groin, place of insertion of cardiac catheter, 24

H

Health care plans, may cover cost of second opinions, 5

Health Resource, Inc. (directory listing), 8

Heart

  damage to, diagnosed by ECG, 17

  echocardiogram of, 32

  exercise and, 33

  nuclear medicine scan of, 45

  viewing in cardiac catheterization, 24

  viewing in coronary angiography, 24

Heart attacks, an example of an emergency, 4

Hospital

  checking with to locate doctors, 8

  medical diagnostic process may be transferred to, 4

  place to have blood drawn, 15

"How To Be a Good Friend To Someone Who's Ill", 75

I

Infection, blood tests used to identify, 15
Injury, many diagnosis begin with, 4
Insomnia. see Sleeplessness
Instinct, what to do if you have negative one
    towards a procedure, 9
Intestine
    see also Large intestine
    barium x-ray of, 20
Intravenous Urography (IVU), description and details, 37-38
Iodine, allergies to, 29, 38
IVU. see Intravenous Urography

J

Job injuries, example of emergency, 4
Johns Hopkins, 9
Joints, endoscopic test for view of, 17

K

Ketones, urine testing for, 14
Kidneys
    CT scan of, 28
    IVU of, 37-38
    ultrasonography of, 51

L

Laboratories, 54-59
    places to have blood drawn, 15
Laparoscopy, description and details, 39

To purchase additional copies of

THE DIAGNOSTIC DILEMMA

visit your local bookstore or

call this toll-free number:

1-800-444-2524